EBM

An Integrated Approach

Akmal El-Mazny

Copyright © 2024 Akmal El-Mazny

All rights reserved.

Amazon KDP, USA

ISBN: 9798329663037

CONTENTS

	PAGE
INTRODUCTION	1
EVIDENCE-BASED MEDICINE (EBM)	
BACKGROUND	2
DEFINITION OF EBM	3
VALUE OF EBM	6
EBM PRACTICE	10
EBM RESOURCES	16
QUALITY OF EVIDENCE	18
GRADES OF RECOMMENDATIONS	20
MEDICAL RESEARCH	
SCIENTIFIC METHOD	22
STUDY DESIGN	23
PARTICIPANTS	27
INTERVENTIONS	30
FOLLOW-UP	31
OUTCOME MEASURES	34
MEDICAL STATISTICS	
DATA MANAGEMENT	35
DESCRIPTIVE STATISTICS	36
ANALYTICAL STATISTICS	46

INTRODUCTION

Evidence-based medicine (EBM) is a systematic approach defined as "the integration of best research evidence with clinical expertise and patient values in direct patient care".

The aims of EBM are to apply the best available research evidence to clinical decision making, and to assess the strength of evidence of the risks and benefits of treatments and diagnostic tests.

In this era of evidence-based health care, both researchers and clinicians need to master EBM in order to critically appraise the medical research, and to judge the implications of reported results.

This book discusses, in an integrated approach, how to practice EBM, the various types of research designs, and the basic process by which medical research and statistics are conducted.

Everything is easy when you know how; hopefully, this book will provide the "know how" for researchers and health-care professionals.

EVIDENCE-BASED MEDICINE (EBM)

BACKGROUND

By the end of the 1970s, a group of clinical epidemiologists led by Prof. *David Sackett*, from McMaster University; Canada wrote a series of articles that were published in the Canadian Medical Association Journal in 1981 under the title of "The Readers' Guide to Medical Literature"; the term "critical appraisal" was used to describe the application of the basic rules of evidence presented in that series.

In 1990, Prof. *Gordon Guyatt*, led by *David Sackett*, introduced the philosophy of medical practice based on knowledge and understanding of the medical literature supporting each clinical decision.

First, he suggested the term "scientific medicine" to describe the new approach but this term was interpreted as being hostile to many practitioners whose practice would be stamped unscientific.

So he proposed another name "evidence-based medicine (EBM)" that first appeared in the autumn of 1990 in an informational document intended for residents applying to the residency program in internal medicine at McMaster University then the term subsequently appeared in print in the ACP Journal Club in 1991; this term afterwards became the standard of medical practice and rapidly invaded the whole world.

DEFINITION OF EBM

EBM is a problem-solving approach in which solutions are sought for questions that arise during clinical practice.

It is defined as "the integration of best research evidence with clinical expertise and patient values in direct patient care" *David Sackett*.

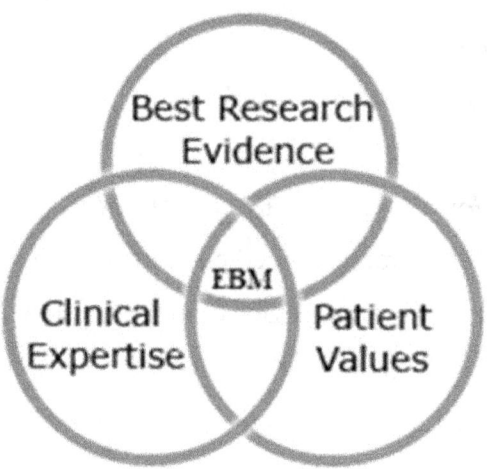

1. Research Evidence

It involves tracking down the best and the latest evidence from research articles that are critically appraised for its validity and usefulness before applying their results to patient care.

EBM helps clinicians to keep their practice up to date and to explain satisfactorily the rationale behind their decisions.

In this way, the clinicians will ultimately provide the best care and outcome to their patients.

Because evidence relies on well-designed research studies to demonstrate the efficacy and effectiveness of diagnostic tests, treatment strategies, new materials and products, the scientific literature is an essential component for "evidence-based practice".

EBM aims for the ideal that healthcare professionals should make "conscientious, explicit, and judicious use of current best evidence" in their everyday practice.

2. Clinical Expertise

It refers to the clinician's cumulated experience, education and clinical skills.

It is important to rapidly identify each patient's unique health state and diagnosis, their individual risks and benefits of potential interventions, and their personal values and expectations.

It is important to emphasize that EBM complements experience and does not replace it.

3. Patient Values

The patient values mean the unique preferences, concerns and expectations each patient brings to a clinical encounter and which must be integrated into clinical decisions if they are to serve the patient.

The practice of EBM is usually triggered by patient encounters which generate questions about the effects of therapy, the utility of diagnostic tests, the prognosis of diseases, or the harms of an intervention.

The full integration of the three components, research evidence, experience and patient's values, into clinical decisions enhances the opportunity for optimal clinical outcomes and quality of life.

Value of EBM

In daily practice the need for valid information about diagnosis, prevention, treatment, prognosis, and harm are growing.

The commonest questions that arise are:
– What is the best diagnostic modality to ask for?
– What is the best treatment should I prescribe?
– What is the prognosis for this patient? or
– What are the harms that might affect this patient from certain treatment or exposure?

The answer for such questions should be based on solid research evidence rather than on opinion, speculations or even past "undocumented and untested" experiences.

However, in reality the answers to these questions usually differ from one clinician to another even in the same institution as clinicians are used to base their decisions on subjective rather than objective standards.

The current prevailing practice among clinicians can be described as the traditional method of medical practice in which clinicians base their decision making process for the daily clinical problems they encounter on their corpus of accumulated medical knowledge and clinical experience.

If they need additional sources, they would try to read about their patient's problem or sometimes they ask for expert's or peers' opinions.

1. Knowledge

Doctors forget what they have learnt and knowledge of best care declines since the year of graduation.

Besides, in 1991, it was estimated that the doubling time of medical knowledge is 19 years.

Probably with the increased amount of scientific research this doubling time has declined to less than 10 years.

This fast pace of increased knowledge coupled with the tendency to forget complicates matters and make access to recent and relevant information more problematic to practicing doctors.

2. Reading

Facing clinical problems, clinicians who usually have a busy schedule and very little time to read, might try to do some readings about their patient problem, but they usually do that in a non-systematic approach; they read a textbook or a journal article that are handy to them.

However, as new knowledge arises textbooks are rapidly outdated and given the huge number of medical journals and articles that are published daily (more than 5000 articles per day), it is difficult, if not impossible, and to find the right and relevant information one is looking for.

3. Experience

Physicians value their experiences; however, studies showed that experienced physicians form a subgroup that needs special attention as there is an inverse relationship between the quality of care provided to patients and the experience of physicians.

Besides, experience is not always helpful especially with new drugs, new treatment modalities and new diagnostic techniques that arise every day without past experience of their use.

4. Experts and Peers Opinions

Experts are frequently wrong as they do not agree together on a given treatment for a given disorder. To choose between variable opinions of experts is mere speculation.

The inconvenience of these traditional methods of medical practice and the exponential increase in the amount of medical information has created a need for a new way of practicing medicine.

This new way of practicing medicine has been called "evidence-based medicine" that has gained much popularity worldwide after the publication of *Gordon Guyatt* and colleagues from McMaster University (Canada) in 1992.

The adoption of an evidence-based approach in medical practice will help clinicians to overcome some of the limitations of the current traditional medical practice.

It will help clinicians to:
- Adopt a lifelong learning process to stay up to date with the current literature.
- Provide the "scientifically proven" current best diagnostic or treatment modality to their patients.
- Rationalize their clinical decision-making process.
- Avoid the pitfalls of the traditional method of medical practice.

EBM Practice

EBM requires the adoption of some new skills including asking clinical questions, basic computer and internet knowledge for electronic searching of the literature and the application of critical appraisal rules in evaluating the clinical literature.

Practicing EBM includes the following steps (5 As Model):

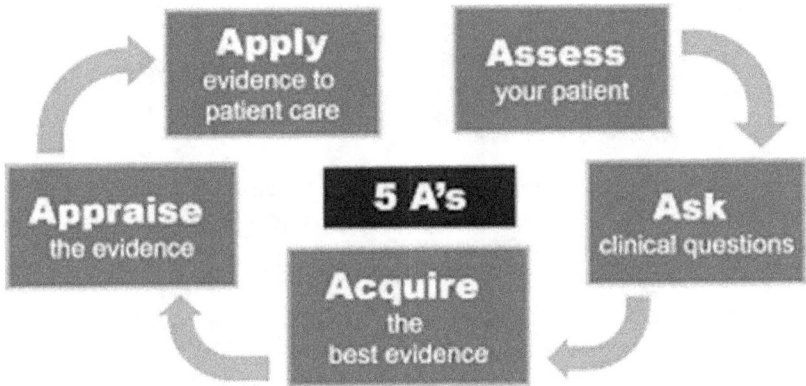

1. Assessment of the Patient

Assessment of the patient is done by:
- History taking,
- Examination and
- Investigations.

Patient's problems will be converted into clinical questions.

2. Asking Clinical Questions

Asking clinical question is to convert the patient's problems into clinical questions in a specific format (PICO format) where:
- P is the problem of the patient,
- I is the intervention or exposure,
- C is the comparison intervention or exposure, and
- O is the outcome the patient looks for (patient-oriented outcome).

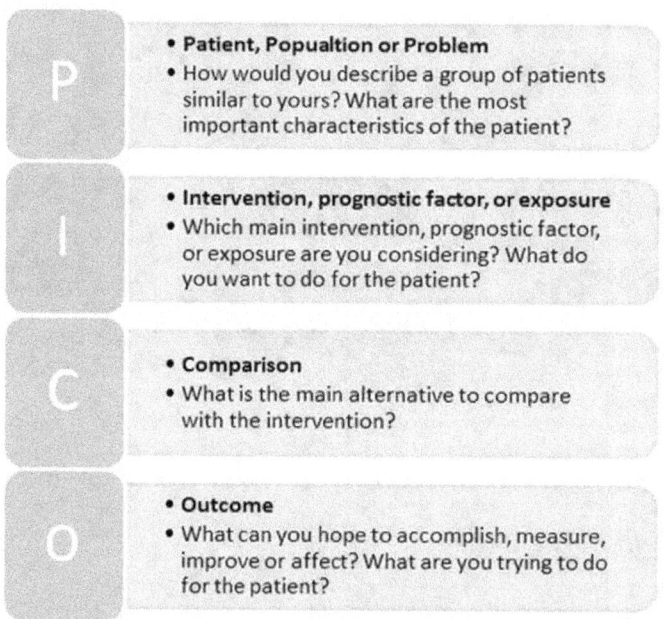

Patient's Problem

This is the description of the group of patients similar to yours or the most important, characteristics of your patient.

This may include the primary problem, disease, or a co-existing condition; sometimes the sex, age (child, adult or elderly) or race of a patient might be relevant to the diagnosis or treatment of a disease.

Intervention

This is the intervention, prognostic factor, or exposure you are considering.

It is something that you want to prescribe or do to the patient (a drug, a test, surgery, or a preventive strategy)

It may also be a factor that may influence the prognosis of the patient (age or a co-existing problem) or an exposure that might affect your patient (asbestos, pollution, cigarette smoking, etc.).

Comparison

This is the main alternative to compare with the intervention; in diagnosis it is a gold standard diagnostic test.

It may be another drug, surgery, no medication or a Placebo.

However, clinical question does not always need a specific comparison.

Outcome

It is something that you hope to accomplish measure, or improve (relief of symptoms, reduce adverse events' improve function, diagnose a disease.

The outcome should be something that matters to the patient (patient-oriented).

3. Acquiring the Best Available Evidence

Acquiring the best available evidence that answers these questions requires an efficient computerized search in EBM resources for finding the best answer (evidence) for the clinical questions generated.

Key words are extracted from the generated PICO question and used in search engines of EBM web sites.

4. Appraisal of the Evidence

Evidence generated from research is not all the same; some evidence is better than others.

Whenever one searches for evidence, he should start looking for the best available one which is obtained from (in descending order):

- Clinical practice guidelines.
- Systematic reviews and meta-analysis.
- Randomized controlled studies.
- Cohort studies.
- Case control studies.
- Case series.
- Case reports.
- Opinions of experts or respected authorities.
- Animal research and in-vitro studies.

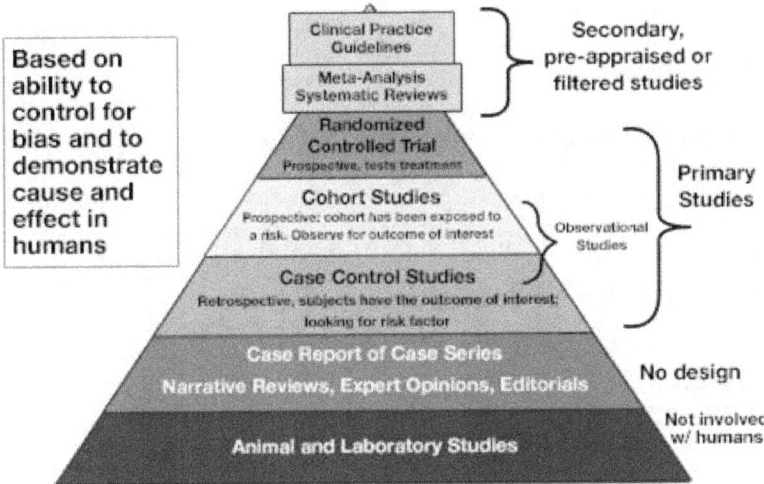

Appraisal of the evidence includes assessment of the relevance and validity of the evidence (clinical applicability).

However, evidence can-be pre-appraised already (as in the Cochrane Library, Clinical Evidence, and the American College of Physicians).

The easiest way for a clinician is to start practicing EBM as an evidence "replicator" who follow evidence-based clinical guidelines, so he does not have to go into steps 3 and 4 (searching and appraising).

Another way of practicing EBM is to be an evidence "user" who can search for readily pre-appraised evidence directly without going into step 4 (appraising).

But with time and practice clinicians would face problems in which there is no readily made evidence to replicate or use; in such circumstances a clinician has to do critical appraisal and practice as an evidence "doer".

5. Applying the Results of the Appraised Evidence

Finally the evidence is integrated with clinical experience and patient values before applying it to the patient.

EBM Resources

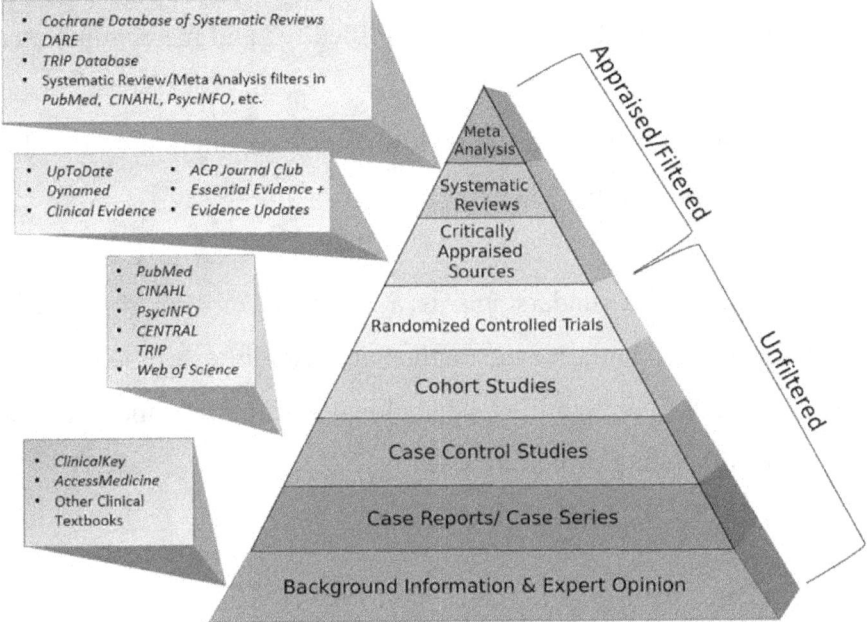

The systematic review of published research studies is a major method used for evaluating particular treatments.

The Cochrane Collaboration is one of the best-known, respected examples of systematic reviews; like other collections of systematic reviews, it requires authors to provide a detailed and repeatable plan of their literature search and evaluations of the evidence.

Once all the best evidence is assessed, treatment is categorized as "likely to be beneficial", "likely to be harmful", or "evidence did not support either benefit or harm".

Generally, there are three distinct, but interdependent, areas of EBM:

The first is to treat individual patients with acute or chronic pathologies by treatments supported in the most scientifically valid medical literature.

The second area is the systematic review of medical literature to evaluate the best studies on specific topics.

Finally, EBM can be understood as a medical "movement" in which advocates work to popularize the method and usefulness of the practice in the public, patient communities, educational institutions, and continuing education of practicing professionals.

QUALITY OF EVIDENCE

Evidence quality can be assessed based on the source type (from meta-analyses and systematic reviews at the top end, down to conventional wisdom at the bottom), as well as other factors including statistical validity, clinical relevance, currency, and peer-review acceptance.

EBM categorizes different types of clinical evidence, and rates or grades them according to the strength of their freedom from the various biases that beset medical research.

Systems to stratify evidence by quality have been developed for ranking evidence about the effectiveness of treatments or screening:

The U.S. Preventive Services Task Force System
- <u>Level I:</u> Evidence obtained from at least one properly designed randomized controlled trial.
- <u>Level II-1:</u> Evidence obtained from well-designed controlled trials without randomization.
- <u>Level II-2:</u> Evidence obtained from well-designed cohort or case-control analytic studies, preferably from more than one center or research group.
- <u>Level II-3:</u> Evidence obtained from multiple time series with or without the intervention.
- <u>Level III:</u> Opinions of respected authorities, based on clinical experience, descriptive studies, or reports of expert committees.

The RCOG System

- <u>Level Ia:</u> Evidence obtained from meta-analysis of randomised controlled trials.
- <u>Level Ib:</u> Evidence obtained from at least one randomised controlled trial.
- <u>Level IIa:</u> Evidence obtained from at least one well-designed controlled study without randomization.
- <u>Level IIb:</u> Evidence obtained from at least one other type of well-designed quasi-experimental study.
- <u>Level III:</u> Evidence obtained from well-designed non-experimental descriptive studies, such as comparative studies, correlation studies and case studies.
- <u>Level IV:</u> Evidence obtained from expert committee reports or opinions and/or clinical experience of respected authorities.

GRADES OF RECOMMENDATIONS

In guidelines and other publications, recommendation for a clinical service is classified by:
- The balance of risk versus benefit of the service, and
- The level of evidence on which this information is based.

The U.S. Preventive Services Task Force System
- Level A: Good scientific evidence suggests that the benefits of the clinical service substantially outweigh the potential risks. Clinicians should discuss the service with eligible patients.
- Level B: At least fair scientific evidence suggests that the benefits of the clinical service outweigh the potential risks. Clinicians should discuss the service with eligible patients.
- Level C: At least fair scientific evidence suggests that there are benefits provided by the clinical service, but the balance between benefits and risks are too close for making general recommendations. Clinicians need not offer it unless there are individual considerations.
- Level D: At least fair scientific evidence suggests that the risks of the clinical service outweigh potential benefits. Clinicians should not routinely offer the service to asymptomatic patients.
- Level I: Scientific evidence is lacking, of poor quality, or conflicting, such that the risk versus benefit balance cannot be assessed. Clinicians should help patients understand the uncertainty surrounding the clinical service.

The RCOG System

- <u>Level A:</u> Requires at least one randomized controlled trial as part of a body of literature of overall good quality and consistency addressing the specific recommendation.
- <u>Level B:</u> Requires the availability of well controlled clinical studies but no randomized clinical trials on the topic of recommendations.
- <u>Level C:</u> Requires evidence obtained from expert committee reports or opinions and/or clinical experiences of respected authorities; indicates an absence of directly applicable clinical studies of good quality.

MEDICAL RESEARCH

SCIENTIFIC METHOD

Scientific research follows a "4-steps approach" known as the scientific method:

1. Observation
Research always starts by an observation.

2. Hypothesis
The observation is used to formulate a research question using the "Null Hypothesis".
"There is no association between 2 variables or 2 groups":

3. Experiment
Each research question has a specific study design to answer:
Therapy --- RCT.
Harm and etiology --- Cohort studies / Case-control studies.

4. Conclusion
Data collected will be statistically analyzed to draw conclusion:
- If the difference between the outcomes did not occur by chance (P value is <0.05), we can reject the null hypothesis.
- If the difference between the outcomes has occurred by chance (P value is ≥0.05), we can accept the null hypothesis.

STUDY DESIGN

It is basic for any researcher to be aware by the different study designs and should always determine the design of the study.

Research can be classified into two main categories:
- Descriptive research and
- Comparative (analytical) research.

The major difference between the two categories is the absence of a control group in descriptive research and the presence of a control group in comparative research.

Descriptive Research

Deals with only one group of patients so comparisons cannot be done and final solid conclusions cannot be drawn from.

1. Case Report

A descriptive research that reports a rare or an unusual disease or a disorder usually in a single patient.

2. Case Series

A research that reports the natural history of a disease or disorder in a group of patients.

3. Prevalence Studies

Describes the prevalence of a certain disease or phenomena.

Comparative (Analytical) Research

Compares between two or more groups, and is further subdivided into two main categories:
– Experimental and
– Observational studies.

While observational studies can be subjected to many types of bias by its nature, experimental studies especially randomized controlled trials are the least design liable to bias.

Thus, randomized controlled trials are the corner stone of EBM and the design that gives the best evidence.

Experimental Studies

The investigators assign the intervention to both the experimental and the control groups.

Simply they, the investigators, are the ones who decide "who takes what?" e.g. they decide who receives the intervention and who receives the placebo or the comparison intervention.

1. Randomized Controlled Trial (RCT)

The investigators assign the intervention to both the experimental and the control groups by chance (at random).

2. Non-Randomized Controlled Trial (Non-RCT)

The investigators did not use random assignment of the intervention to the experimental and the control groups.

Observational Studies

According to their relation to time, observational studies are further sub-classified into cohort, case-control, and cross sectional studies.

1. Cohort Study

A research that starts with two groups one is exposed to a certain exposure and the other is not (control group) and both groups are followed up forward in time till the occurrence of the outcome.

2. Case-Control Study

A research that starts with the outcome (a group of patients having a certain disease and another disease-free control group) and looks backward in time (either by recalling the history of exposure or looking for the exposure in the hospital records).

3. Cross-Sectional Study

A research that compares between two groups in the same moment in time without either backward recall or forward follow-up.

The following chart shows the basic study design types:

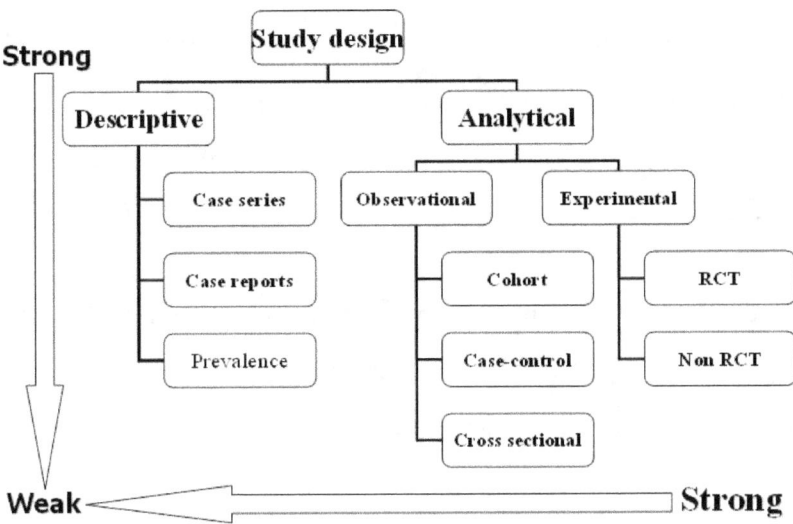

The following diagram shows the basic types of observational studies according to their relation to time:

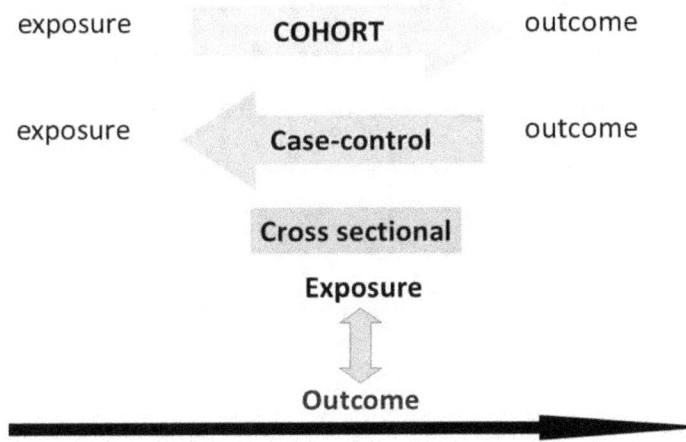

PARTICIPANTS

You must have clear description of your study participants (previously known as patients, subjects or cases):

Inclusion Criteria

- Clear definition of the included participants' characteristics.
- Clear definition of the included pathology.
- Clear definition of the presentation.

Exclusion Criteria

All individuals with any confounding characteristics should be excluded from the study participants.

Confounders are non-study variables that may affect the outcomes of the study; e.g. diabetes is a confounder when you study treatment of moniliasis because diabetic cases are more resistant to monilia treatment than non-diabetic cases.

Control Group

Contrary to what is usually believed, the size of the control group should be at least equal to that of the cases groups and better to be larger.

Controls are sometimes problematic because there may be no way to recruit them simple in the study; this will take much effort to search for such suitable individuals without biasing the study.

You should explain clearly the size, characteristics and sources of the control group especially if the controls are normal healthy individuals.

Group Assignment in Clinical Trials

In all clinical trials, you should describe how did you allocated the study participants into groups.

It is well known that randomized trials are much more powerful than non-randomized ones.

If you performed a randomized trial, you should describe:
– The method of randomization used (coin toss, dice rolling, sealed envelopes or random number table),
– Who did randomization, and
– How this randomization is concealed.

Long Scenario

Many of the journals now request a flow chart to show the participants track line throughout the study.

The following flow chart shows the scenario of enrolling the participants in the study:

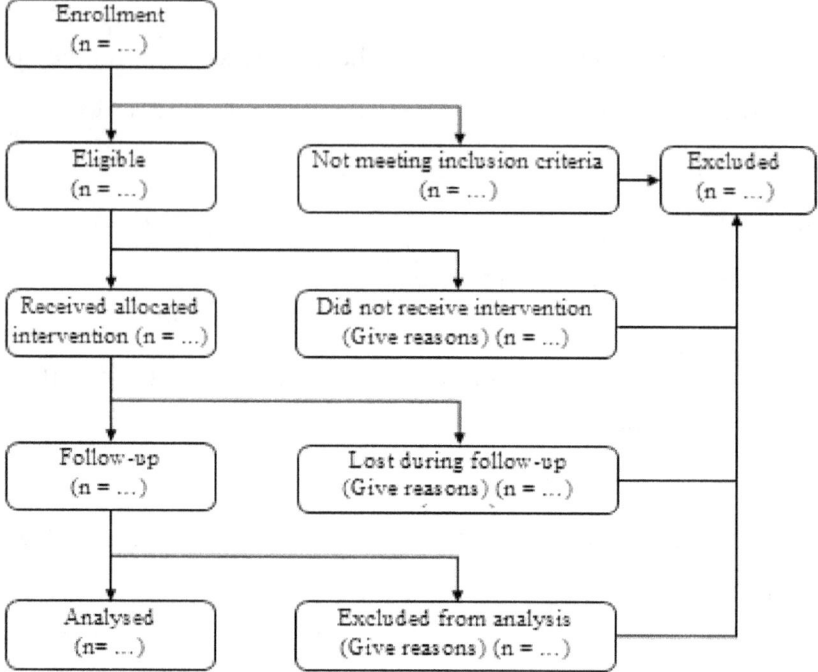

INTERVENTIONS

This part starts usually by reporting the human rights committee approval, ethical committee approval, consent or explanation; this may be the first part in the subjects and methods.

Important basic signs and special investigations are first described briefly to include or exclude cases and as preliminary to study investigations.

Study Investigations
- Enough details of tools, machines, instruments and kits (trade name, model, source, and contact data).
- Specify critical values.
- Specify effect size needed to be found.
- Old techniques are briefly described with references.
- Modifications of standard techniques are fully described with methodology references.

If you did something unusual or used an unfamiliar method, you must explain.

If you are giving placebo in a clinical trial, you must describe how the study drug cannot be differentiated from placebo.

Follow-up

For how long?
- Your follow-up must be enough to cover all study outcomes.

What was done?
- Follow-up investigations should be complete and efficient to evaluate all possible outcomes.

What interval?
- The interval of the follow-up should be adjusted to record all possible changes in the course of all the studied outcomes.

Blinding

Blindness is ensuring that a person remains unaware of the type of intervention a subject has been allocated to until the end of the study.

If possible, both the patients and the observers should be blinded to the given treatment; this makes better results especially if the outcome is opinion based.

It is important to decrease tendency to report more favorable outcomes in the control group, and less favorable outcomes in the control group; and to decrease bias in measuring outcome by investigators (ascertainment bias).

Types of Blinding

- Single blinded: Blinding the subjects participating in the trial.
- Double blinded: Blinding the subjects and investigators (clinicians, interviewers, laboratory personnel).
- Triple blinded: Blinding the subjects, investigators and committee responsible for monitoring outcome as well as persons who perform data entry, analysis and statistics.

Types of Bias in RCTs

- Selection bias: Improper patient selection and allocation to treatment groups.
- Ascertainment bias: Bias in recording and analyzing data.
- Dropout bias: Mishandling of patients who drop-out the study.
- Publication bias: Publishing only trials with positive and ignoring those with negative results.

Dropouts

The longer the follow up, the higher the dropout participants; it is logic to think that dropouts will affect the validity and power of the study.

Although there is no universally accepted cutoff, a dropout of 20% of participants will considerably affect the study.

So, you should, as much as possible, report how many the dropouts in your study and why they are dropped out.

It is a common practice to exclude dropouts as they represent missing data and analyze the rest of participants (called "per-protocol analysis").

This may be accepted in descriptive or observational studies (although still will affect the validity and power); yet it is never accepted in clinical trials because it may lead to overestimation of the treatment effect which is very dangerous in such type of research.

Intension to Treat Analysis

This means that all participants will be analyzed as they were randomized whether completed the study or dropped out.

Advantages
− Preserves randomization.
− Bias in the conservative direction.

Disadvantages
May lead to underestimation of the treatment effect, however, this is safer for the patient.

Worst Case Scenario

All dropouts from the study group will be considered bad outcomes, and all dropouts from the control group will be considered good outcome.

OUTCOME MEASURES

Every researcher should clearly state the outcomes of the research; outcomes may be:

Primary Outcome(s)

These are the principal outcome(s) of the research; e.g. example: treatment of anovulation; treatment of osteoporosis.

The researcher should always choose patient oriented outcomes rather than disease oriented outcomes; e.g. in a research about treatment of anovulation, pregnancy is a patient oriented outcome while ovulation is a disease oriented outcome; in a research about treating osteoporosis, frequency of fractures is a patient oriented outcome while bone mineral density is a disease oriented outcome.

Secondary Outcome(s)

These are other outcomes than the principal one(s); e.g. the primary outcome in a research may be success of certain treatment for certain disease.

However, the research also studies side effects and complications, patient compliance, cost, etc. as secondary outcomes.

MEDICAL STATISTICS

DATA MANAGEMENT

- Collection of data (results of observations).
- Organization, summarization and description of data (Descriptive Statistics).
- Analysis of data to draw statistical conclusions and make statistical decisions (Analytical Statistics).

Statistics

- The science concerned with data management.
- The science of measuring uncertainty.
- The science of measuring the known sources of variation.
- The art of drawing correct conclusions from inaccurate data.

DESCRIPTIVE STATISTICS

Statistical methods that summarize a large set of data into a few meaningful numbers.

Classification of Data
– Numerical (quantitative) data.
– Categorical (qualitative) data.

Numerical (Quantitative) Data

Data that are basically represented in numbers such as age, weight, height, temperature, blood pressure, etc…

Characteristics of Quantitative Data
– Numerically represented.
– Accurate representation of data.
– All mathematical rules can be correctly applied.
– Analyzed by the most powerful statistical methods.

Distribution of Data

To draw the mostly correct conclusions by statistics, you must determine how frequent each value had occurred in the studied data "distribution".

STATISTICS - DESCRIPTIVE

Determination of data distribution is an important requirement to do correct statistics.

When a graph is drawn to show the frequency of occurrence of each value in a data set, this is called data distribution graph (histogram).

If most of data are in the middle range and the extreme values are equally rare, the shape of the curve will be symmetrically bell shaped; this is called the "normal distribution".

Otherwise it is called "non-normal distribution".

Normally distributed data are analyzed using what is known as "parametric tests".

Non-normal data are analyzed using "non-parametric tests".

Parametric statistics is generally more powerful than non-parametric statistics in making decisions and conclusions and should always be used whenever possible.

Non-normal data can be made normal by what is known as "data transformation".

The most famous method of transformation is calculating the log values.

Normal

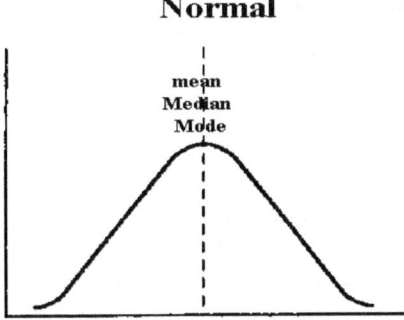

Rt Tailed (Skewed Rt or +ve skew)

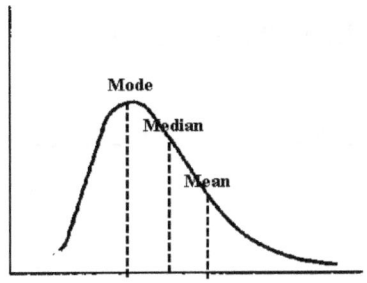

Lt Tailed (Skewed Lt or -ve skew)

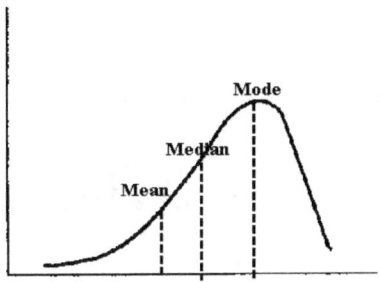

Data Distribution

Description of Numerical Data

- Measures of central tendency (location)

    Mean

    Median

    Mode

- Measures of variation (dispersion)

    Standard deviation

    Range

- Frequency distribution

I. Measures of Central Tendency (Location)

These are values that represent the middle or midpoint of the possible values of a variable.

The most famous measures of central tendency are:

1. The Mean

It is the arithmetic average of a set of numerical data.

It represents the central value of the data that depends on the size of the data values.

It is calculated by dividing the sum of the data values by number of data.

It is most suitable for normally distributed quantitative data especially of large number of records.

In data with few records or many extreme values (outliers) the use of arithmetic mean is of low value.

2. The Median

It is the middle value of a ranked array (it divides the array into 2 equal parts).

If the total number of series values is even, the median is the arithmetic mean of the 2 middle values.

It is of special importance in non-normal quantitative data, and data with many outliers.

3. The Mode

It is the most frequently occurring value.

Some series have no mode while others have more than one mode.

It must be equal to one or more value in the data set.

II. Measures of Variation (Dispersion)

Describe the data variations around the central measure.

1. The Variance and Standard Deviation

Variance is the mean of squared deviation around the mean.

It represents an index of the spread of measurements around the mean.

It describes subject – to – subject variation within the data array.

It is more sensitive than the range because it is affected by every value in the data set.

It is not practical because the deviation is squared, so to be practical, its value should be square rooted which gives the "standard deviation (SD)" which is most suitable with the arithmetic mean.

A range of one SD above and below the mean (abbreviated to ± 1 SD)
± 1 SD includes 68.2% of the values.
± 2 SD includes 95.4% of the values.
± 3 SD includes 99.7% of the values

Coefficient of Variation

It is the parentage of SD: mean ratio (SD ÷ mean × 100).

It has the advantages of nullifying the effect of the unit of measurement of the variable.

2. The Range

Most suitable with the median.

It is the difference between the maximum and minimum values; sometimes the range may be calculated between 2 reference values not the maximum and the minimum.

When the range is between the 1st and 3rd quarters of the data it is called the interquartile range.

III. Frequency Distribution

If we transformed numerical data into categories, it is possible to describe through frequency tables.

Each row in the table represents a "class" and the range of the class is called the "class interval"; ideally, the class interval should be equal.

Categorical (Qualitative) Data

Data not represented basically in numbers such as sex, race, blood groups, hair color, etc…

Characteristics of Qualitative Data
- Less accurate representation of data (depends on estimation rather than measure).
- Mathematical rules cannot be correctly applied.
- Analyzed by less powerful statistical methods.

Classification of Qualitative Data

1. Nominal Data

Data which can be categorized but with no specific order (not ranked) e.g. sex, color of hair, race, religion, blood groups, etc…

Dichotomous data are type of nominal data the result of which may be one of 2 responses e.g. occurrence of pregnancy, menopausal status, etc.

Polychotomous data are those with more than 2 responses e.g. blood group A, B, AB, or O; white, black, yellow, oriental race, etc…

2. Ordinal Data

Ordered (ranked) data e.g. severity scale (mild, moderate, severe); tumor stages, scoring systems, etc.

Description of Categorical Data

Categorical data can be described as:
- Number
- Fraction
- Percent

Frequency is the number of times of the occurrence of an event.

Relative frequency is the number of times of the occurrence of an event as a fraction (or percent) of the total.

Cumulative frequency is the fraction (or percentage) of observations that are less than the upper limit of each interval.

Frequency measures are the only way to describe categorical data and are used to describe numerical data when transformed into categories.

The 2×2 frequency table formed of only 2 columns and 2 rows (the totals are not counted).

Statistical Inference and Confidence Interval (CI)

Although we cannot know the true population parameters using any sample, it is possible to calculate a range or an interval in which we will be confident that the true population parameters lie inside.

This concept is called "statistical inference" and the interval is called the "confidence interval (CI)".

This interval can be calculated from one single done sample.

Calculation of the CI depends on calculating the amount of change of the estimate from sample to sample, this is called the standard error (SE) and this, in turn, depends on the amount of variation in the sample and the sample size.

Thus, the higher the variation in the done sample (e.g. SD) the higher the SE and the smaller the sample size, the higher the SE and vice versa.

A last point; this CI is actually estimated, how much can I trust this interval in including the true population parameter?

There is a general agreement that 95% confidence is enough and a 5% error will not affect the statistical results.

ANALYTICAL STATISTICS

1. Statistical Comparison

Statistical comparisons aim to detect if sample difference is significant (associated with population difference) or non-significant (not associated with population difference and is due to chance).

The answer lies in the *p* value (probability of chance) that will result from the statistical test whatever is.

The *P* (Probability) Value

There is a general agreement that if the probability of chance is <0.05 (*P* value <5%) we can safely conclude that the difference is real and not due to chance.

If the *P* value is 0.05 or more, we can conclude that the difference is due to chance.

We can also formulate the original question in another way; we can assume that there is no difference between the groups and then ask whether this assumption is right or wrong.

The assumption of "no difference" is called the "null hypothesis" (the hypothesis of no difference, H_0) and we ask whether the H_0 is true or false.

If the P value is <0.05, this means that the probability of chance is low, thus the difference is significant, thus we can reject the null hypothesis and H_0 is false.

If the P value is ≥0.05, this means that the probability of chance is considerable, thus the difference is non-significant, thus we accept the null hypothesis and H_0 is true.

The lower the P value, the less likely it is that the difference happened by chance and so the higher the significance of the finding.

Which test I choose?

The following chart shows the basic concept of choosing comparison tests:

Numerical	2 groups	Normal	Student's t test
		Non-normal	Mann-Whitney U test
	> 2 groups	Normal	ANOVA test
		Non-normal	Kruskall Wallis test
Categorical	Frequency ≥ 5		Chi-square ($\chi 2$) test
	Frequency < 5		Fisher exact test

2. Correlation and Regression

Sometimes you notice that in two series of quantitative or ordinal data, the values of one variable may vary correspondingly with the other one.

For example, it is well known that as age increases in children, the height increases as well, also, in old age as age increases the bone mineral density decreases as well; this relation is called "correlation".

When the two variables increase and decrease in parallel (same direction), this called "positive correlation".

If one variable goes and the other goes down proportionally (opposite directions), it is called "negative correlation".

Graphically, correlation is represented by what is known as the "scatter diagram".

In this diagram, each individual is represented by a dot that represents the values of the correlated variables; one variable is put on the X axis, and the other is put on the Y axis.

When the points on the scatter diagram represent a linear pattern, the correlation is termed "linear correlation" while if taking a curvilinear pattern it is "non-linear correlation".

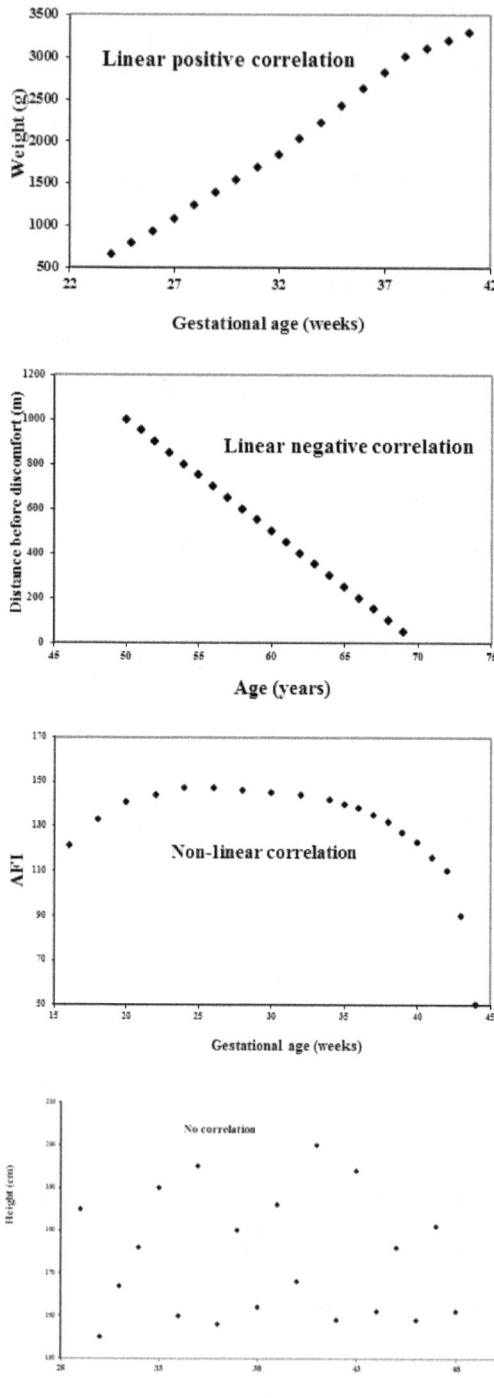

Correlation Studies

In normally distributed data, linear correlation is tested using the "Pearson's product moment correlation" method that depends on the calculation of the correlation coefficient "r".

The range of r is from 0 (means no correlation) to 1 (means perfect relation).

The "algebraic sign" means the direction of correlation and is not a value.

The following is a good rule of thumb when considering the size of a correlation:
$r = 0$–0.2: very low and probably meaningless.
$r = 0.2$–0.4: low correlation that might warrant further investigation.
$r = 0.4$–0.6: reasonable correlation.
$r = 0.6$–0.8: high correlation.
$r = 0.8$–1.0: very high correlation; check for errors or other reasons for such a high correlation.

This guide also applies to negative correlations.

In non-normally distributed data, correlation is tested using the "Spearman rank correlation" method which depends on calculating the correlation coefficient (ρ).

Regression

Regression is a method used to derive an equation to estimate the value of one variable when the value of another correlated variable (or variables) is known.

If the equation includes two variables only, it is called "simple regression", while if there are more than two variables it is called "multivariable or multivariate or multiple regression". If one variable is binary, the regression model is called "logistic regression".

The graphic representation of regression is like correlation uses the scatter diagram with addition of a straight line representing the regression equation line; it is called the "trend line" or "regression line".

This line is passing on the maximum number of pints and is nearest to all points; thus every set of data will have a special trend line.

The regression coefficient gives the "slope" of the graph, in that it gives the change in value of one outcome, per unit change in the other.

This regression equation can be applied to any regression line; it is represented by: $y = a + bx$

To predict the value "y" (value on the vertical axis of the graph) from the value "x" (on the horizontal axis), "b" is the regression coefficient and "a" is the constant.

Correlation and regression are generally needed when there is one variable difficult to measure and another one easy to measure.

If both variables are correlated, we can use the easy measured variable to estimate the value of the difficult to measure variable.

Correlation measures the strength of the association between variables.

Regression quantifies the association; it should only be used if one of the variables is thought to precede or cause the other.

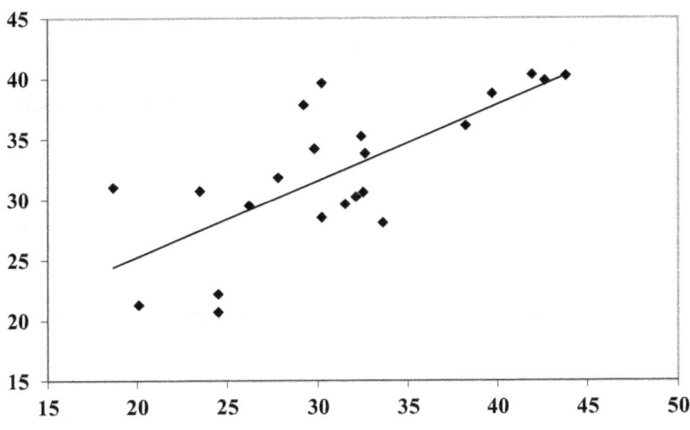

Regression Line

3. Sensitivity and Specificity

To calculate the accuracy of the new diagnostic test, a sample of individuals is exposed to both the new test and a suitable gold standard.

According to the results of the gold standard, the participants are divided into diseased and non-diseased.

While according to the results of the new diagnostic test, the participants are divided into test positive and negative.

True +ve
Are cases diagnosed +ve by the new test and proved to be diseased by the gold standard.

True -ve
Are cases diagnosed -ve by the new test and proved to be non-diseased by the gold standard.

False +ve
Are cases diagnosed +ve by the new test but proved to be non-diseased by the gold standard.

False -ve
Are cases diagnosed -ve by the new test but proved to be diseased by the gold standard.

How Accurate is the Test?

Sensitivity

It is the proportion of diseased individuals who are diagnosed +ve by the new test (true +ve).

Sensitivity = true +ve / all diseased cases in the study (which is true +ve + false -ve).

Specificity

It is the proportion of non-diseased subjects who are diagnosed -ve by the new test (true -ve).

Specificity = True -ve / all non-diseased cases in the study (which is true -ve + False +ve).

Overall Accuracy

It is the proportion of those who were truly diagnosed in the study to the total number.

Overall accuracy = (True +ve + true -ve) / (all subjects).

Does the Patient Have the Disease or Not?

Although sensitivity and specificity have been used for a long time to evaluate the accuracy of new diagnostic tests, yet they are not useful to evaluate the usefulness of the test in helping a particular patient.

Suppose that the patient has a positive (or a negative) test, the question to be answered is not how much accurate is the test but the question that the patient needs an answer to is "given this test result; what is my probability of having the disease?"

These indices are known as the predictive values:

Positive Predictive Value (PPV)

It is the probability of a patient with a positive test to have the disease.

PPV = true +ve / all +ve.

Negative Predictive Value (NPV)

It is the probability of a patient with a negative test to be free of the disease.

NPV = true -ve / all –ve.

Unfortunately the predictive values of a test are not constant as they depend on the prevalence of the disease in the population, i.e. they change with the increase or the decrease of the prevalence.

In other words they change with the pre-test probability of the disease as prevalence is considered the probability of having the disease.

The Likelihood Ratio

From the above it is clear that what is important in helping a particular patient is how much the test is able to change our minds from what we thought before the test (pre-test probability) to what we think afterward (post-test probability).

The diagnostic tests that produce big changes from pretest to post-test probabilities are the important tests and likely to be useful to us in our practice.

The new practical way to express the usefulness of a diagnostic test is calculating the likelihood ratios of positive test (LR +ve) and of negative test (LR -ve).

The Likelihood Ratio of a Positive Test (LR +ve)

LR +ve = Sensitivity / (100 - specificity).

The more is the LR +ve the better is the test to increase the probability of the presence of the disorder.

LR +ve = 1 means no use of the test (no change between the pretest probability and posttest probability).

The Likelihood Ratio of a Negative Test (LR -ve)

LR -ve = (100 - sensitivity) / Specificity.

The less is the LR -ve the better is the test to decrease the probability of presence of the disorder.

LR -ve = 1 means no use of the test (no change between the pretest probability and posttest probability).

The likelihood ratios are used with the pretest probability to determine the posttest probability.

www.ingramcontent.com/pod-product-compliance
Lightning Source LLC
Chambersburg PA
CBHW071959210526
45479CB00003B/999